Alkaline Ketogenic
GREEN SMOOTHIES

Creamy & Delicious, Low-Carb, Low Sugar Green Smoothie Recipes for Weight Loss, Beauty and Health

By Elena Garcia
Copyright Elena Garcia © 2020

Sign up for new books, fresh tips, super healthy recipes, and our latest wellness releases:

www.YourWellnessBooks.com

All rights reserved. No part of this publication may be reproduced, stored in a retrieval system, or transmitted, in any form or by any means, electronic, mechanical, photocopying, recording or otherwise, without the prior written permission of the author and the publishers.

The scanning, uploading, and distribution of this book via the Internet or via any other means without the permission of the author are illegal and punishable by law. Please purchase only authorized electronic editions, and do not participate in or encourage electronic piracy of copyrighted materials.

Disclaimer

A physician has not written the information in this book. It is advisable that you visit a qualified dietician so that you can obtain a highly personalized treatment for your case, especially if you want to lose weight effectively. This book is for informational and educational purposes only and is not intended for medical purposes. Please consult your physician before making any drastic changes to your diet.

All information in this book has been carefully researched and checked for factual accuracy. However, the author and publishers make no warranty, expressed or implied, that the information contained herein is appropriate for every individual, situation or purpose, and assume no responsibility for errors or omission. The reader assumes the risk, and full responsibility for all actions and the author will not be held liable for any loss or damage, whether consequential, incidental, and special or otherwise, that may result from the information presented in this publication.

The book is not intended to provide medical advice or to take the place of medical advice and treatment from your personal physician. Readers are advised to consult their own doctors or other qualified health professionals regarding the treatment of medical conditions. The author shall not be held liable or responsible for any misunderstanding or misuse of the information contained in this book. <u>The information is not intended to diagnose, treat, or cure any disease.</u> It's merely an inspiration to live a healthy lifestyle.

If you suffer from any medical condition, are pregnant, lactating, or on medication, <u>be sure to talk to your doctor</u> before making any drastic changes in your diet and lifestyle.

Contents

Introduction 8
Alkaline Keto Green Smoothies- Food Lists 12
    Recommended Alkaline Keto Fruit 12
    Recommended Alkaline Keto Greens 13
    Alkaline Keto Friendly Vegetables 15
    Alkaline Keto Spices & Herbs for Your Smoothies 17
    Alkaline Keto Sweeteners and Supplements (Optional) 18
    Alkaline Keto Fats 19
    Alkaline Keto Nuts and Seeds 20
    Alkaline Keto Friendly Milk & Other Liquids to Use in Smoothies 21
    Why Alkaline Ketogenic Smoothies? How Can They Help Us? 23
    WHAT IS THE ALKALINE DIET? 27
    Your Wellness Books Email Newsletter 37
About the Recipes-Measurements Used in the Recipes 38
    Recipe#1 Green Dream Weight Loss Smoothie 40
    Recipe#2 Chlorophyll Spanish Gazpacho 42
    Recipe#3 Healing Celery Smoothie 43
    Recipe#4 Immune System Energy Smoothie 44
    Recipe#5 Seducing Bullet Proof Creamy Green Smoothie 45
    Recipe#6 Keto Indulgent Creamy Aroma Smoothie 46
    Recipe#7 Creamy Green Relaxation Smoothie 47
    Recipe#8 Double Your Energy Smoothie 48
    Recipe#9 Ketoricious Energy Smoothie 49
    Recipe#10 Herbal Wellness Smoothie 50
    Recipe#11 The Supermodel Glow Smoothie 51
    Recipe#12 Quick Detox Smoothie Soup 52

Recipe#13 Simple Anti-Inflammatory Alkaline Keto Mix 53

Recipe#14 Green Mineral Coconut Balancer.. 54

Recipe#15 Cucumber Creamy Green Smoothie 55

Recipe#16 Boost Your Brain Smoothie 56

Recipe#17 Spice Up Your Health Smoothie.. 57

Recipe#18 The Anti-Age Smoothie 58

Recipe#19 Refreshing Radish Green Smoothie 59

Recipe#20 Cilantro Oriental Alkaline Keto Smoothie 60

Recipe#21 Vitamin C Alkaline Keto Green Power 61

Recipe#22 Green Mineral Comfort Smoothie Soup 62

Recipe#23 Green Fat Burner Smoothie 63

Recipe#24 Massive Green Power Plants Smoothie 64

Recipe#25 Easy Guacamole Smoothie.. 65

Recipe#26 Cucumber Kale Alkaline Keto Smoothies 66

Recipe#27 Sexy Flavored Spinach Smoothie 67

Recipe#28 Spicy Broccoli Smoothie..68

Recipe#29 Bullet Proof Chai Tea Anti-Inflammatory Green Smoothie ... 70

Recipe#30 Easy and Tasty Green Smoothie Maravilla ... 71

Recipe#31 Green Vegan Keto Smoothie for Weight Loss ... 72

Recipe#32 Quick Unwind Smoothie ... 73

Recipe#33 Spicy Mediterranean Protein Smoothie ... 74

Recipe#34 Vitamin C Energy and Mood Boosting Smoothie ... 75

Recipe#35 Green Almond Protein Hormone Balancer ... 76

Recipe #36 Creamy Alkaline Smoothie Refresher ... 77

Recipe#37 Alkaline Keto Fill Me Up Smoothie ... 78

Recipe#38 Holistic Beauty Smoothie ... 79

Recipe#39 Heal Up Smoothie ... 80

Recipe#40 Create Massive Balance Alkaline Smoothie ... 81

Recipe#41 Simple Detox Spicy Smoothie ... 82

Recipe#42 Ultimate Wellness Alkaline Green Smoothie ... 83

Recipe#43 Liver Cleanse Green Smoothie ... 84

Recipe#44 Super Antioxidant Green Smoothie ... 85

Recipe#45 Keto Fill Me Up Smoothie ... 87

Recipe#46 Hormone Rebalancer Sweet Veggie Smoothie ... 88

Introduction

Ready to discover the new (and still underground) way of making smoothies?

If your goal is to enjoy more energy, live a healthy lifestyle and (if desired) lose weight – you have come to the right place!

Alkaline Keto style of making green smoothies is one of the best wellness tools you could possibly get into.

Here's why...

Alkaline Keto Green smoothies are:

-very low in sugar (because they focus on fruits and veggies that are naturally low in sugar)

-dairy and soy-free (we use alkaline-keto friendly plant-based or nut milk instead!)

-naturally gluten-free (by going gluten-free, or at least reducing gluten in your diet, you will be able to think clearly, and you will feel so much lighter!)

-Super low carb, but still very filling (perfect for weight loss diets)

-Rich in good fats for sustainable energy!

-Rich in mind-body energizing chlorophyll to help you look and feel amazing!

-You will not feel hungry on those smoothies...

Alkaline Keto Green Smoothies - Introduction

Our smoothies are jam-packed in vital nutrients, vitamins and minerals – to help you stay healthy and have beautiful, glowing skin and strong hair.

Rich in healthy, plant-based protein – so that your body can thrive, inside out.

Vegan, paleo, and keto friendly!

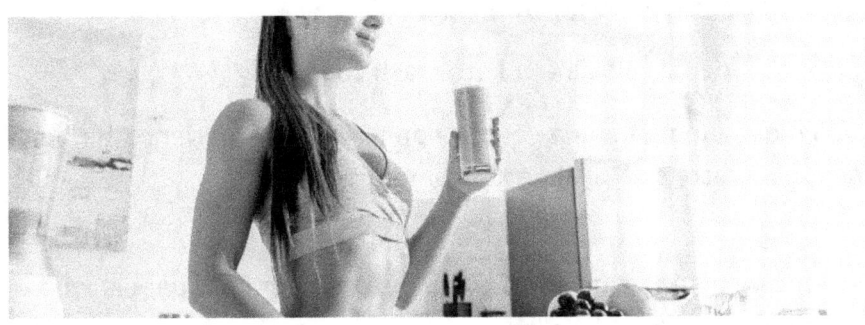

They are just perfect to help you:

-enjoy more energy

-stay full for hours

-get you closer to your weight loss, health and fitness goals!

The best part?

-you don't need any fancy ingredients

-the recipes are beginner friendly

-you can enjoy a variety of taste – naturally sweet – sour – or even spicy smoothies

-you can easily make the recipes even on a busy schedule

-most recipes can be used as a meal replacement

Included are:

-simple food lists/shopping lists

-extra tips and guidance (even if you are new to alkaline-keto, or green smoothies – we got you covered)

-beginner friendly alkaline & keto crash course

-SOS motivation – to help you stay on track and experience all the incredible results of alkaline keto smoothies

This recipe book is a practical guide designed for busy people who value their health and wellbeing.

I am very excited to have you onboard, so let's get started!

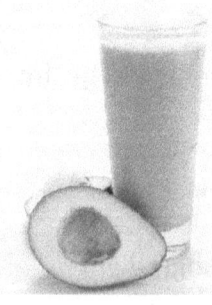

Alkaline Keto Green Smoothies - Introduction

What I really like about alkaline-keto smoothies is that unlike traditional smoothies they don't use any high sugar fruit.

That makes them perfect for people who need to follow low-sugar, low-carb diets.

Another benefit is that they can be easily turned into delicious creamy soups (served raw or slightly cooked). You can easily customize your alkaline keto soups by adding in some protein of your choice to enjoy a satisfying, nutritious meal. The recipes contained in this book will show you how. Alkaline Keto Green Smoothies are much more than just smoothies!

Finally, the recipes, as well as "nutritional philosophies" contained in this book, are very flexible and open-minded. Anyone can benefit from them; they are not only for people who follow alkaline or keto diets. So, whether you are alkaline keto full-time, or merely part-time (you are looking for easy tips and recipes to improve your health), you have come to the right place!

I believe that just by creating a simple health habit of making one big alkaline keto green smoothie a day, you have the power to transform your body and health.

The moment you decide to focus on abundance and enriching your diet with nutrient-packed, fresh foods (healthy foods that do not contain any nasty chemicals, sugars or crappy carbs) you will automatically crave all the good stuff.

So, without any further ado, let's do this. I am so excited for You!

Alkaline Keto Green Smoothies- Food Lists

Recommended Alkaline Keto Fruit

Both alkaline, as well as ketogenic diets, encourage you to stay away from sugar, including fruit that is high in sugar.

However, low-sugar fruits are allowed, and there are many ways to make them taste delicious (the recipes will show you how).

It's all about balance!

Alkaline Keto Approved Fruits for Green Smoothies

- Limes
- Lemons
- Grapefruits
- Avocado (yes, it's a fruit)
- Tomato (yea, it's a fruit)
- Pomegranate

The following fruit is also allowed in small amounts, to add to taste:

- Blueberries
- Sour cherries
- Raspberries
- Strawberries
- Other berries
- Green apple (sparingly)

Recommended Alkaline Keto Greens

All leafy greens are alkalizing and detoxifying to your body. They are also compatible with the keto diets, and since this is a green smoothie book, they are our main guest here!

- Spinach
- Kale
- Microgreens
- Swiss Chard
- Arugula
- Endive
- Romaine Lettuce

+ other fresh leafy greens and greens as well as:

- Parsley
- Mint
- Chive
- Dill

Quick Green Tip for Busy People:

I prefer fresh greens to green powders...but...whenever I go traveling, or I am really pressed for time, I use a delicious green powder blend called Organifi.

I also like to add it to my recipes as it makes my smoothies taste really nice while adding a ton of superfoods at the same time.

This green powder is naturally sweet and is a great addition to my green smoothies and juices.

You can learn more about it and how I use it with my recipes on my website (treat it as an additional recommendation to help you save your time on research).

You will also find other resources from reputable health experts, such as keto for people over 40, 50, and 60, an alkaline cleanse to quit sugar, and awesome customized keto plans, I have successfully used on my path to wellness and weight loss:

www.yourwellnessbooks.com/resources

Now, back to our food lists....

Alkaline Keto Friendly Vegetables

Yes, I know, I know. Not very sexy...

Most people don't like veggies. I am not judging, I used to be one of them!

I was never a fan of raw veggies. But, they can taste really delicious in smoothies. So even, if you are not a veggie person, don't worry. You can do this.

Trust me, your body will be grateful!

Who knows, maybe eventually you will feel motivated and inspired enough to start your day with a big alkaline-keto, veggie-packed green smoothie?

As you will later see, we will be using some awesome spices and creamy nut and plant-based milk, so everything will taste delicious.

Besides, as you dive deeper into smoothies, your taste buds will get used to them, and eventually you will be craving veggies. But, if you're still new to this, don't worry. Rome wasn't built in a day.

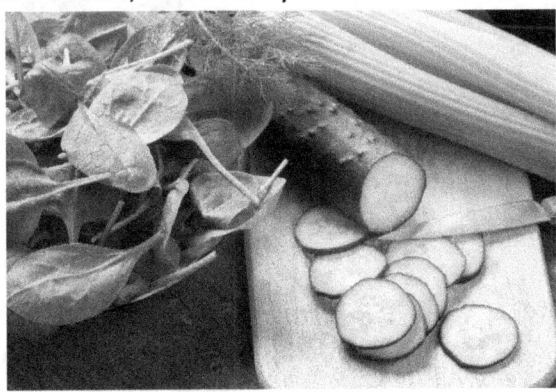

Alkaline Keto Green Smoothies - Introduction

All veggies have one thing in common...
They are both alkaline and keto friendly. Why?

Because they are naturally low in sugar. At the same time, they are full in nutrients, low carb and naturally gluten-free.

Alkaline diet loves low-sugar fruits and veggies and so does the keto diet. All the veggies are very alkaline-forming to the body (more on that later) and they can also be used on the keto diet.

They taste amazing in smoothies, especially red and green peppers.

Your alkaline -keto veggie list to use in your green smoothies:

- Red bell pepper
- Green bell pepper
- Yellow bell pepper
- Zucchini
- Broccoli
- Asparagus
- Colliflower
- Garlic
- Onion
- Cucumbers
- Radishes
- Artichokes

Alkaline Keto Green Smoothies - Introduction

Alkaline Keto Spices & Herbs for Your Smoothies

The following herbs and spices will make your smoothies taste delicious. Real game changer if you ask me!

Alkaline Keto spices and herbs are also full of anti-inflammatory properties.

Again, since there are no sugars and no nasty carbs, the following herbs and spices are both alkaline and keto friendly.

- Cinnamon
- Himalaya Salt
- Curry
- Red Chili Powder
- Cumin
- Nutmeg
- Italian spices
- Oregano
- Rosemary
- Lavender
- Mint
- Chamomile
- Fennel
- Cilantro
- Moringa

Herbs and spices are great for all kinds of healthy smoothies!

From naturally sweet, to sour or spicy.

Get used to using spices and you will never get bored with your green smoothies.

Alkaline Keto Sweeteners and Supplements (Optional)

This one is very important, because we want to stay away from all forms of sugar, as much as possible.

However, if you like sweet, or need something to help you transition away from sugar, don't worry.

Your transformation doesn't have to be healthy.

Stevia is very helpful if you want to make a sweet smoothie without using sugar or sugar-containing foods or supplements.

If you are looking for natural supplements to optimize your alkaline keto green smoothies and make them even more nutritious, you can also try:

- Green Powders
- Moringa Powder
- Maca Powder
- Ashwagandha Powder

Again, these are all optional. However, if you are interested in learning more, please visit our private website where I share more complimentary info with my readers. I have listed my favorite brands, green powders, and other health supplements to help you save your time:

www.YourWellnessBooks.com/resources

Alkaline Keto Fats

Plant-Based

(these are both alkaline and keto friendly)

- Olive oil (organic, cold-pressed)
- Avocado oil
- Hemp oil
- Flaxseed oil
- Coconut oil
- Sesame oil

Please note, there is no need to purchase all of them, one, or two is enough; my two favorites are coconut oil and olive oil.

***Wellness tip – whenever your body craves sugar, have 1 tablespoon of coconut oil.

It always does the trick for me!

Then, you feel back on track and you can proceed to making a nutrient-packed alkaline keto green smoothie with good oils to keep sugar cravings away for good!

Alkaline Keto Nuts and Seeds

These taste amazing in smoothies and will help you stay full for hours.

- Almonds (In moderation as they are richer in carbs)
- Cashews (in moderation as they are richer in carbs)
- Brazilian Nuts
- Macadamia Nuts
- Walnut
- Pine
- Pistachio
- Hazelnut
- Chia seeds

Of course, if you have any nut allergies, skip them in your smoothies.

I have noticed that chia seeds work for most people (even those allergic to almonds or cashews), but, be sure to follow your own agenda, and talk to your health practitioner if needed.

Alkaline Keto Friendly Milk & Other Liquids to Use in Smoothies

Plant-Based

(these are both alkaline and keto friendly)

- Almond milk
- Coconut milk
- Hazelnut milk
- Coconut water
- Herbal infusions
- Organic Apple Cider Vinegar

+ coffee and caffeine, in moderation (caffeine is not considered alkaline, and overdoing caffeine is not very keto either, bit again, moderation is key).

If you have any questions about the food lists/ingredients for alkaline keto green smoothies, please email me at:
info@yourwellnessbooks.com

You can also sign up for our free newsletter at:

www.yourwellnessbooks.com/email-newsletter

and then reply to my first email and say hi.

Please note, the lists I have shared are basic food lists to make alkaline keto friendly smoothies because I want to keep it as simple as possible.

But they are not set in stone. I am always happy to answer your questions regarding the ingredients you want to use in your smoothies.

Now, let's move on to the next part!

Why Alkaline Ketogenic Smoothies? How Can They Help Us?

The problem is that most people eat way too many carbs and sugars. The temptations are everywhere, I know! To make it even worse, we eat processed carbs and sugars (pasta, candy, cakes, etc.). Most people find it hard to start their day without carbs and sugar.

Luckily, once you get into the alkaline ketogenic lifestyle, through adding more low carb, low sugar, high-fat green smoothies into your diet, you will be able to experience a whole range of health and wellness benefits as well as possible prevention of many diseases.

Low carb, low sugar diets are proven to:

-manage your sugar levels, prevent diabetes

-normalize your hormones and auto-immune system

-improve your neurological health

-has even been used in clinical settings to prevent Alzheimer's, epilepsies, type 3 diabetes

Here are other benefits of aligning your dietary choices with an alkaline ketogenic-friendly way:

-you will experience reduced hunger and reduced cravings

-you will be burning fat and reducing carbs and so normalizing your insulin levels

-you will protect your heart while raising the good cholesterol

-you will enjoy the anti-age benefits, as keto foods promote longevity and vitality (while nobody ever promised us we will live forever, by making a decision to stay healthy, we make sure that the time we are here on earth, we feel good and are vibrant).

Your transformation starts right here, right now.

Alkaline Keto smoothies are one of the best and easiest tools to help you get started, even if you are busy.

Now, let's have a look at:

1. What the keto diet actually is.
2. What the alkaline diet is.
3. How these two can be successfully combined for optimal benefits while respecting your nutritional lifestyle choices and preferences.

The goal of this book is simple- I don't want to "push" any specific kind of a diet bandwagon or make you feel bad for eating a certain way.

Instead, I want to inspire you and give you simple, healthy, and delicious tools (alkaline ketogenic smoothies) to help you get closer to your health, wellness, and fitness goals every day.

How about setting one simple goal, to begin with? Make 1 alkaline ketogenic smoothie a day? Take meaningful I and inspired action from a place of curiosity and empowerment, not fear.

Forget about perfection and focus on progress...

We are very, very close to help you get started. In fact, if you have already read my book *Alkaline Ketogenic Mix*, or *Alkaline Diet for Weight Loss and Wellness*, or *Alkaline Paleo Mix*, feel free to skip the following section and dive right into the recipes.

What really matters here is practice. But a little bit of inspiring information and learning more about our amazing bodies can also help.

So...

WHAT IS THE KETO DIET?

The simplest definition is:

The ketogenic diet is a diet low in carbs and high in healthy fats.

It encourages to massively reduce the carbohydrate intake and replace it with good, healthy fats (more on healthy vs. unhealthy fats later). This cutback in carbs puts your body into a metabolic state called ketosis.

When in ketosis, your body becomes super-efficient at burning fat for energy. A ketogenic diet can also help reduce blood sugar and insulin levels.

The fact is that we are designed to have periods where we "fast from carbs" and when our glucose levels are depleted.

Then, we start using our body very cleverly, using ketones for fuel. Ketones are the result of our body burning fat for food. The liver converts body fats and ingested fats into ketones.

Transition your diet into a more keto-friendly diet, it's straightforward. It means fewer sugars and carbs and more good fats while eating well!

Following this simple rule (even without going keto full-time) will help you transform your health. It will also help you lose weight naturally if you stay committed to it.

You will no longer be hooked on all those "crappy carbs" and with the new "keto energy" you will feel much more motivated to work out and be more active.

So, here's what the ketogenic diet consists of:

-75%- 80% fat (don't worry, it's all good fat and will not make you fat).

-5-15% healthy, clean protein

-5% good, unprocessed carbs (yea, you can still eat some carbs and the carbs we will be focusing on, will be healthy unprocessed no sugar carbs so no worries, there is no starvation involved here).

While it may seem like something hard to follow, especially when you still got that pasta meal on your mind, it will all become effortless after you get into the creamy, fatty, and actually guilt-free ketogenic friendly smoothie recipes!

WHAT IS THE ALKALINE DIET?

"Going green" is the way to describe an alkaline diet and lifestyle because the focus is on green vegetables in general, as they are the most alkaline food you can ingest.

The benefits of the alkaline diet are numerous. Let us name a few:

WEIGHT LOSS

An alkaline diet will assist you in losing weight. One way that it does this is obvious. The foods you will be eating are very healthy, rich in minerals and low calorie in general.

You will also be reducing the amount of acid in your body. The body stores fat to protect itself from an abundance of acid. It is a self-preservation method. This is part of the reason why people who exercise a lot and drink an excess of caffeine cannot seem to lose those extra pounds. Their bodies are clinging to that fat to minimize the effects of all of the acid in their systems. Caffeine is really acid-forming, and it's not the most sustainable source of energy. That is why we recommend you drink it in moderation, for your own occasional enjoyment rather than a source of energy you depend on.

Another benefit of an alkaline lifestyle regarding weight loss is that alkaline systems have more oxygen in their cells. Oxygen is a very essential part of eliminating fat cells from the body. The more oxygen in your system, the more efficient your metabolism will be.

ENERGY

Going green does not only give you energy for the apparent reason that you are eating many more healthy, energizing vitamins. You are negating the acid-induced lethargy that is brought on by an unhealthy acid-forming diet.

Not only do our bodies need an abundance of oxygen to lose weight, but we also need oxygen in our cells to energize us. The lack of oxygen in our cells causes fatigue. No, it is not just because you worked too late or partied to hard the night before. It is internal. If your cells are trying to function in a highly acidic environment, they will not be able to transfer oxygen efficiently; leading of course to exhaustion.

Cells in the body also make something that is called adenosine triphosphate (ATP). If your system is very acidic, it harms the ability of your cells to produce it. In the scientific world, it is known as the "energy currency of life." The ATP molecule contains the energy that we need to accomplish most things that we do (both internally and externally).

BODILY FUNCTIONS

Another benefit of the alkaline lifestyle is that your body will be able to function at an optimum level instead of being inhibited by acids:

- Your heartbeat is thrown off by acidic wastes in the body. The stomach suffers greatly from over-acidity.

- The liver's job is to get rid of acid toxins, but also to produce alkaline enzymes. By simply reducing your acid intake, you can internally boost your alkalinity thanks to your liver!

- Your pancreas thrives on alkalinity. Too much acid in your system throws off your pancreas. If you eat alkaline foods, your pancreas can regulate your blood sugars.

- Your kidneys also help to keep your body alkaline. When they are overwhelmed by an acidic diet, they cannot do their job

- The lymph fluids function most efficiently in an alkaline system. They remove acid waste. Acidic systems not only have a slower lymph flow causing acids to be stored; they can also cause acids to be reabsorbed through lymphatic ducts in your intestines that would typically be excreted.

MENTAL FOCUS

The alkalinity of the system is one of the best ways to focus and strengthen the mind. Just as the rest of the body is poorly affected by acid-forming foods and other toxins, so is your brain. And as we all know, it should be possible to control your emotions and decision making with your mind. Guess what? If your body is too acidic and is not alkaline, your mental clarity will be cloudy, your decision making could be off, as well as your emotional state.

DETOX

Another huge benefit of an alkaline lifestyle is detoxification. First, you are going to be cutting out processed foods that are continually adding toxins to your system.

Secondly, you are going to be eating foods that allow your body to detox and rid itself of the acids that have built up in your system all this time. When we detoxify our bodies, our emotions, bodily functions, and mental functions can operate at their optimum levels.

The number of benefits that come with living alkaline are numerous. As you help your body rebalance its optimal blood pH, you will find, as we did, that you have never felt better. We are still seeing improvement and reaping the rewards of this holistic approach to not only eating alkaline foods but living alkaline.

Alkaline vs. Acidic? Sounds like the title fight for a lightweight boxing match. In reality, it is a fight, a fight for the pH balance of your body. pH levels are basically the measure of how acidic a liquid is.

Our bodies function optimally when our blood is at about 7.35 - 7.45 pH.

pH levels range from 0 to 14. 0 is the highest level of acidity, but basically, everything 0-7 would be considered acidic. The 7-14 range is alkaline.

Before we dive into complicated pH discussions, here is one thing to understand:

-The alkaline <u>diet is not about changing or "raising" your pH</u>. This is where many alkaline guides go wrong. You see, our body is smart enough to **self-regulate** our pH for us, no matter what we eat.

Unfortunately, when you constantly bombard your body with acid-forming foods (for example processed foods, fast food, alcohol, sugar, crappy carbs, and even too much meat) you torture your body with incredible stress. Why? Well because it has to work harder to maintain that optimal pH...

Here's simple example...

Imagine you immerse yourself in a bath filled with ice. You say, but hey, my body can self-regulate its optimal temperature, right? And yes, it can. But it will eventually collapse, and you will get ill. The same happens with nutrition and our blood pH.

You can spend years indulging in toxic, processed, acid-forming foods that only deprive your body of its vital nutrients, saying: "But hey, my body will self-regulate its optimal blood pH."

And again, it will...but sooner or later it will give up and manifest a disease. It will accumulate fat as its natural defense function to protect your body from over-acidity. We don't wanna end up there, right?

So, to sum up- the alkaline diet is a natural, holistic system, a nutritional lifestyle that advocates the consumption of fresh, unprocessed foods that are rich in nutrients. These are called alkaline foods, and they help your body stimulate its optimal healing functions. Yes! A healthy body needs nutrients, and fresh fruits and vegetables are great for that.

The problem is that nowadays, most diets are filled with acid-forming foods that eventually make it hard for the body to regulate its optimal, healthy blood pH. Acidosis is very common in this day and age thanks to things we drink as well: coffee, alcohol, sugar, crappy carbs, and sodas all have an acidic effect on our bodies. Not to mention the chemicals many people take in through things like smoking and drugs (even prescription drugs have this effect).

There are many ways that you could become acidic. Eating acid-forming foods, stress, taking in too many toxins, and bodily processes all cause acidity in the body. Our internal systems try to balance themselves out and bring pH up with the help of alkaline minerals that we can ingest through our diet. If we do not take in a higher percentage of alkaline than acidic foods, we can become too acidic.

When you are acidic, it makes every process that your body does typically much more difficult or impossible for it to accomplish. We cannot absorb the beneficial nutrients we need from our food correctly. Our cells are not able to produce energy efficiently.

Our bodies are not able to fix damaged cells properly. We will not be able to detoxify properly. Fatigue and illness will drag you down. Sounds horrible; does it not? Here are some signs that you are overly acidic:

- ✓ Feeling tired all the time. You have no physical or mental drive at all.
- ✓ You always feel cold.
- ✓ You get sick easily.
- ✓ You are depressed or just feel "blah" all the time for no real reason
- ✓ You are easily overstimulated and stressed by noise, light, etc.
- ✓ You get headaches for no apparent reason
- ✓ You get watery eyes or inflamed eyelids.
- ✓ Your teeth are sensitive and may crack or chip
- ✓ Your gums are inflamed, and you are susceptible to canker sores

- ✓ You have recurring bouts with throat problems including tonsillitis

- ✓ Acidic stomach with acid indigestion and reflux is always an issue

- ✓ Your fingernails crack, split, and break

- ✓ You have super dry hair that sheds and is hay-like with split ends

- ✓ You have dry, ashy skin

- ✓ Your skin breaks out in acne or is irritated when you sweat

- ✓ You get leg cramps and spasms (this includes restless leg syndrome).

(Of course, remember that whenever you experience any health/medical conditions, you need to see your doctor first and get a checkup.)

Changing your diet to one that is full of alkaline foods is one of the easiest and best things you can do for your overall health. I was so ecstatic that I did! And the best thing is- we will be combining alkaline foods with keto friendly meals to make it easy, delicious and fun! Much simpler to follow for the long term.

But the way we see it is this- it's perfect! Plus, it's not a diet, it's a lifestyle.

What I really like about the alkaline diet is that you don't have to be 100% perfect. It's enough to make sure you add a ton of greens and veggies and make your diet rich in alkaline foods.

It's easy to do when you focus on serving your lunch or dinner with a big green salad or start drinking alkaline keto smoothies (I will show you how to go about it in the recipe section later).

When it comes to the alkaline diet, there is something called the 70/30 rule meaning that about 70% of your diet should be fresh, nutrient dense alkaline-forming foods and the remaining 30% can be acid- forming foods (however they still should be clean and organic, for example, grass-fed meat or organic eggs).

The common mistakes with the ketogenic diets:

The most common mistake that people make is that they do not include enough veggies with their keto animal-based foods. That can cause imbalance and acidity. Hence, I am such a big fan of keto and alkaline diets combined together. Green vegetables are a fantastic addition to your keto diet.

They will help you have more energy and also add more variety to your diet.

The real keto lifestyle is about variety, abundance, and energy. It's hard to be successful with a keto diet if a menu consists entirely of animal products.

The role of alkaline foods

It's essential to get a ton of greens and alkaline foods as these foods are rich in minerals and vitamins while at the same time don't contain sugar.

I have been promoting alkaline foods for years.

They oxygenate your body and help you have more energy and can be combined with other diets such as paleo or keto diet.

In its optimal design, alkaline diet advocates using good plant-based oils such as avocado and olive oil, and coconut oil and it also excludes wheat products and crappy carbs.

Foods that are rich in sugar are also excluded. The alkaline diet includes low sugar fruits (limes, lemons, grapefruits, etc.)

One of the main principles of the alkaline diet is adding a ton of green veggies into your diet.

The best way to be adding these alkaline foods is via low sugar and low carb alkaline keto smoothies! And you are already learning how to do that.

The Role of Chlorophyll

Most people think they are doing great by adding a little bit of iceberg lettuce to their lunch...

While this can be an amazing step forward, it's not enough. A little salad here and there is not enough to balance out our acidic lifestyles (stress, pollution, allergens everywhere).

The solution?

Chlorophyll. Heck, this is why I am writing this book. More and more people need to turn to green smoothies for help.

But, of course, traditional green smoothies with their overload of high-sugar fruit may not be enough...

So, let's have a look at the benefits of chlorophyll. This will be your SOS motivation. Whenever you feel like you're getting off track, or you feel like skipping your green smoothie, be sure to re-read this page.

Prevention is easier than cure, trust me on that one, I had to learn it the hard way. But the good news is that baby steps are not so hard.

Don't overcomplicate the process in your mind. Your mind should be your friend, your ally, not your enemy!

The benefits of consuming chlorophyll-rich foods and drinks:
1. Beautiful, healthy-looking, glowing skin.
2. Can reduce inflammation.
3. Stimulates natural body detox, so that your body can get rid of toxins that can lead to imbalances and illness.
4. Can stimulate weight loss (as the body no longer needs to store fat to counterbalance acids).
5. Can act as a natural deodorant and reduce bad breath.

Your Wellness Books Email Newsletter

Before we dive into the recipes, we would like to offer you free access to our VIP Wellness Newsletter

www.yourwellnessbooks.com/email-newsletter

Here's what you will be receiving:
-healthy, clean food recipes and tips delivered to your email
-motivation and inspiration to help you stay on track
-discounts and giveaways
-notifications about our new books (at massively reduced prices)
-healthy eating resources to help you on your journey

No Fluff, no spam. Only excellent and easy to follow info!

Sign up link (copy this link to your phone, tablet, or PC):

Problems with signing up? Email us at:
info@yourwellnessbooks.com

www.yourwellnessbooks.com/email-newsletter

About the Recipes-Measurements Used in the Recipes

The cup measurement I use is the American Cup measurement.

I also use it for dry ingredients. If you are new to it, let me help you:

If you don't have American Cup measures, just use a metric or imperial liquid measuring jug and fill your jug with your ingredient to the corresponding level. Here's how to go about it:

1 American Cup= 250ml= 8 Fl.oz.

For example:

If a recipe calls for 1 cup of almonds, simply place your almonds into your measuring jug until it reaches the 250 ml/8oz marks.

I hope you found it helpful. I know that different countries use different measurements, and I wanted to make things simple for you. I have also noticed that very often those who are used to American Cup measurements complain about metric measurements and vice versa. However, if you apply what I have just explained, you will find it easy to use both.

Alkaline Keto Green Smoothie Recipes

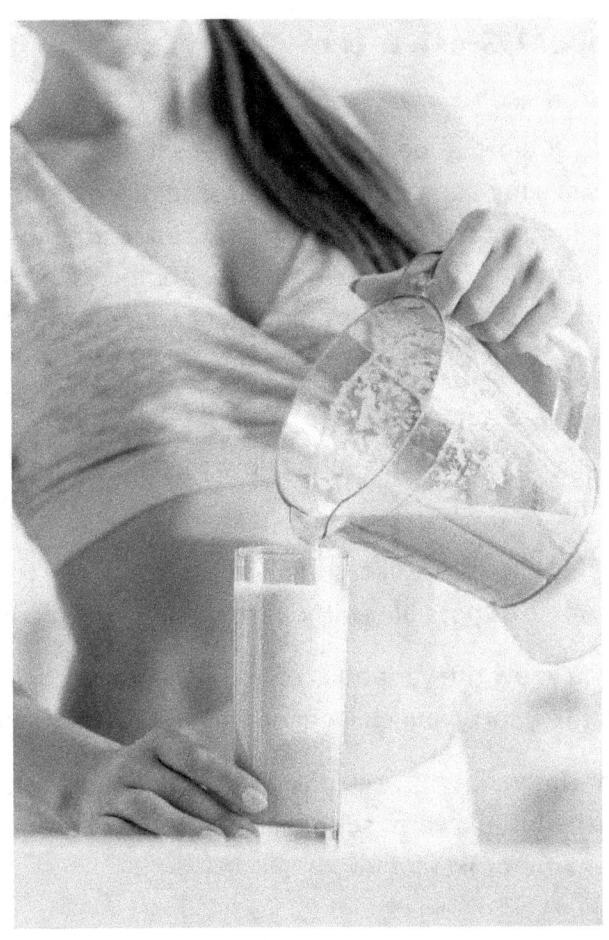

Recipe#1 Green Dream Weight Loss Smoothie

This green vegetable smoothie blends the best of the alkaline and keto worlds. It's my number one recommendation if your goal is weight loss. It may take some time to get used to green vegetable smoothies. Especially if you are more accustomed to drinking "sweety-carby-fruity" smoothies (not that good for you, unfortunately).

But trust me, after a few green smoothies, and fantastic energy they provide, you will be wondering how you could ever live without them.

Himalaya salt really makes it taste delicious. Now, I like to keep my recipes as simple as possible, without too many ingredients.

But to let you know the variations of this recipe- you could also add in some cilantro, curry and chili pepper if you like spicy smoothies.

If you go for this variation, you may also heat up the smoothie and serve it as a beautiful, warm soup (and add some coconut or other full-fat cream on top). Enjoy!

Servings: 2

Ingredients:

- 1 cup coconut or almond milk (unsweetened)
- 1 cup water (filtered, preferably alkaline)
- 1 small avocado, peeled and pitted
- A handful of spinach
- 1 tablespoon coconut oil or flaxseed oil
- Pinch of Himalaya salt to taste

Instructions:

1. Place all the ingredients in a blender.

2. Blend well.
3. Serve and enjoy!

Recipe#2 Chlorophyll Spanish Gazpacho

This recipe is a variation of the original Spanish gazpacho recipe in a super alkaline keto green version.

Serves: 2

Ingredients

- 3 medium sized cucumbers, peeled and chopped
- 1 green bell pepper
- 1 big garlic clove, peeled
- 2 tablespoons extra-virgin, cold pressed olive oil
- 1 tablespoon of avocado oil
- 1 cup filtered water
- Half cup almond milk
- Pinch of Himalayan salt
- Pinch of black pepper

Instructions

1. Place all the ingredients in a blender and process until smooth.
2. Serve in a smoothie glass and enjoy!
3. If you prefer to enjoy this recipe as a soup, you can garnish it with some chopped veggies, herbs and spices.
4. Enjoy!

Recipe#3 Healing Celery Smoothie

Here comes another delicious veggie smoothie recipe.

Celery is a very alkaline forming ingredient. It is rich in vitamin C, fiber, alkaline minerals such as potassium and is also very hydrating and replenishing.

Perfect for a simple, green super alkaline smoothie.

Serves 1-2

Ingredients

- ½ cup of celery
- 1 tablespoon virgin, cold pressed olive oil
- Pinch of Himalayan salt
- 1 teaspoon of raw cashews
- 1 cup coconut vegan yoghurt, unsweetened
- 1 small avocado
- Pinch of black pepper to taste
- A few fresh cilantro leaves to garnish

Instructions

1. Place all the ingredients in a blender and process until smooth.
2. If needed season with Himalayan salt and black pepper.
3. Serve in a smoothie bowl or glass and garnish with some fresh cilantro leaves.

Recipe#4 Immune System Energy Smoothie

This is a super simple alkaline green smoothie that will help you boost your immune system by enriching your diet with vitamin C and a myriad of alkaline minerals.

Serves 1-2

Ingredients

- 2 big limes, peeled
- 1 cup of coconut or almond milk
- A handful of kale leaves, washed
- Optional- a few drops of liquid chlorophyll
- 1 lime wedge to garnish (1 per serving)
- 1 tablespoon coconut oil
- 1 teaspoon cinnamon powder
- Stevia to sweeten, if needed

Instructions

1. Place in a blender.
2. Process until smooth.
3. Serve in a smoothie glass and garnish with a wedge of lime.
4. Enjoy!

Recipe#5 Seducing Bullet Proof Creamy Green Smoothie

This smoothie is called "seducing" for a reason.

It is perfect early in the morning to help you concentrate at work. It combines the antioxidant properties of blueberries with good fats and a bit of coffee.

While you don't want to end up in a position where you depend on caffeine, using it in small amounts to optimize your performance while nourishing your mind and body with a ton of alkaline nutrients will be very helpful! I love this smoothie for my long writing sessions.

Servings: 1-2

Ingredients:

- 1 strong expresso (use organic, quality coffee)
- 1 cup thick coconut milk
- 1 big avocado
- 1 tablespoon chia seeds or chia seed powder
- Half teaspoon of any green powder of your choice
- 2 tablespoons coconut oil

Instructions:

1. Blend all the ingredients.
2. Pour your smoothie into a smoothie glass and serve with ice cubes if needed.
3. Enjoy!

Recipe#6 Keto Indulgent Creamy Aroma Smoothie

This recipe is very nutritious and it can also be served as a quick, raw, or almost raw soup (you can add some eggs or protein to make it more filling).

Healthy lifestyle doesn't have to be difficult or time-consuming.

Servings: 2

Ingredients:

- 1 cup thick coconut milk (full fat)
- 2 tablespoons coconut oil
- Half avocado, peeled and sliced
- Half lemon, peeled and sliced
- 1 cup fresh parsley leaves, washed
- Half teaspoon Himalaya salt
- 2 tablespoons fresh cilantro leaves
- Black pepper (optional)

Instructions:

1. Place all the ingredients in a blender.
2. Process until smooth.
3. Serve and enjoy!
4. If needed season with some black pepper.

Recipe#7 Creamy Green Relaxation Smoothie

This smoothie uses healing herbal infusions such as chamomile and rooibos.

Chamomile is famous for its sleep and calm-inducing properties, while rooibos is full of alkaline ingredients. It's also naturally sweet, and so is this smoothie.

Servings: 2-3

Ingredients:

- 1 cup rooibos tea (cooled down, use 1 teabag per cup)
- 1 cup chamomile tea (cooled down, use 1 teabag per cup)
- 1 small avocado, peeled and pitted
- 1 small lime, peeled and sliced
- Half cup thick coconut milk
- 2 tablespoons coconut oil
- 1 teaspoon any green powder of your choice, or a few liquid chlorophyll drops
- A handful of cashews
- Stevia to sweeten if needed

Instructions:

1. Place all the ingredients in a blender.
2. Process until smooth.
3. Enjoy now or place in a fridge for later.

Recipe#8 Double Your Energy Smoothie

This smoothie is can be served as a quick lunch to help you double your energy and feel amazing. No more afternoon energy crashes!

Serves 1-2

Ingredients

- 1 cup of fresh dairy-free vegan yogurt or full fat coconut milk
- Half cup water, filtered, preferably alkaline
- 2 cucumbers, peeled and chopped
- Half an avocado, peeled and pitted
- 1 cup iceberg lettuce
- A pinch of Himalayan salt to taste
- A pinch of black pepper to taste
- 1 tablespoon coconut oil
- A handful of raw cashews

Instructions

1. Place all the ingredients in a blender.
2. Process until smooth.
3. Taste to see if you need to add some salt.
   Serve in a bowl and sprinkle over some black pepper. Enjoy!

Recipe#9 Ketoricious Energy Smoothie

This recipe uses hemp oil, which is great to re-balance hormones, soothe anxiety and improve the mood.

Serves 1-2

Ingredients

- 1 tablespoon of hemp oil
- 1 cup coconut milk
- 1 avocado, pitted and peeled
- A handful of cilantro leaves, washed
- 1 teaspoon spirulina
- Pinch of Himalayan salt
- Pinch of curry powder
- Optional (if you like it spicy) a pinch of chili powder

Instructions

1. Place all the ingredients in a blender.
2. Process until smooth.
3. Taste to check if you like to taste or if you need to add a bit more of Himalayan salt or curry powder
4. Serve in a smoothie glass, or a bowl and enjoy!

Recipe#10 Herbal Wellness Smoothie

This smoothie is great for digestion and relaxation.

It also helps prevent sugar cravings.

Serves 1-2

Ingredients

- 1 tablespoon of mint leaves
- 2 tablespoons of coconut oil
- ½ cup of cashew milk
- ½ teaspoon of fresh vanilla
- ½ cup chamomile infusion, cooled

Instructions

1. Place cashew milk, mint leaves and vanilla in a blender.
2. Process until smooth.
3. Pour into a smoothie glass and mix it with chamomile infusion (warm or cold, depending on your preferences).
4. Enjoy!

Please note – cashew milk can be replaced with almond milk, coconut milk, or any nut or plant based milk of your choice. Just make sure there is no added sugar.

Recipe#11 The Supermodel Glow Smoothie

Good fats from avocado and coconut oil will help you stay full longer and prevent sugar cravings. It will help you have a glowing, healthy looking skin too! All this while helping your body get back to balance.

Serves 1-2

Ingredients

- 1 tablespoon coconut oil
- 1 cup of cashew or other nut milk of your choice
- 2 small zucchini, steamed and peeled
- 1 big tomato
- Handful of fresh cilantro leaves, washed
- 1 teaspoon moringa powder

Instructions

1. Place all the ingredients in a blender.
2. Process until smooth.
3. Pour into a smoothie glass, stir well, serve and enjoy!

Recipe#12 Quick Detox Smoothie Soup

This smoothie will help you enrich your diet with healthy, alkalizing vegetables. I like to make this smoothie in the evening and use one serving as a quick detox soup (yea, you can heat it up a bit) and then I keep the second serving as a quick morning smoothie.

Servings: 2

Ingredients:

- 1 green bell pepper
- 1 small avocado, peeled and pitted
- 1 small garlic clove, peeled
- Pinch of black pepper and chili
- 1 cup water (filtered, or alkaline water)
- 1 tablespoon extra-virgin olive oil
- Himalaya salt to taste

Instructions:

1. Place all the ingredients in a blender.
2. Process until smooth, serve, and enjoy!

Recipe#13 Simple Anti-Inflammatory Alkaline Keto Mix

This smoothie is perfect if your goal is to have more energy and reduce inflammation.

Good fats will help you stay full and focused for hours. Maca powder is optional here. Personally, I love it!

Servings: 1-2

- 1 cup fresh almond milk, unsweetened
- Half cup water, filtered, preferably alkaline water
- 2-inch turmeric, peeled
- A handful or arugula leaves
- Half avocado, peeled and pitted
- 1 tablespoon coconut oil
- Stevia to sweeten (optional)

Instructions:

1. Blend all the ingredients in a blender.
2. Serve and enjoy.
3. This drink is great first thing in the morning. But you can also sip on it during the day to enjoy more energy.

Recipe#14 Green Mineral Coconut Balancer

This delicious smoothie uses stevia (both alkaline and keto friendly natural sweetener) so that you can enjoy an excellent, creamy sweet taste.

It also uses maca powder, which is a hormone re-balancer for women.

Enjoy!

Ingredients:

- 1 cup coconut milk, unsweetened
- 1 big avocado, peeled and pitted
- A few drops of liquid chlorophyll, or half teaspoon of Organifi or other green powder of your choice
- 1 tablespoon coconut oil
- A bit of stevia to sweeten
- Half teaspoon fresh maca powder

+ a few lime slices and ice cubes to serve if needed

Instructions:

1. Place all the ingredients in a blender.
2. Process until smooth.
3. Serve and enjoy!
4. This smoothie also tastes delicious when chilled or half frozen.

Recipe#15 Cucumber Creamy Green Smoothie

This is one of my favorite "on the go" smoothie recipes as it doesn't require that many ingredients.

Thanks to cucumbers, It's full of alkaline minerals and very hydrating.

Servings: 2

Ingredients:

- 2 big cucumbers, peeled and roughly sliced
- 1 cup full-fat coconut milk (unsweetened)
- Pinch of Himalaya salt to taste
- Pinch of black pepper to taste
- 6 radishes, sliced
- 2 tablespoons chive, chopped

Instructions:

1. Place the cucumbers, and coconut milk in a blender.
2. Add the Himalaya salt and black pepper.
3. Blend well and pour into a smoothie glass or a small soup bowl.
4. Add in the radishes and chive.
5. Mix well and add more Himalaya salt and black pepper if needed.
6. Sprinkle the cheese and enjoy!

Recipe#16 Boost Your Brain Smoothie

The flaxseed meal is an excellent source of Omega-3 fatty acids, aka "good fats". After having this smoothie, not only will you feel full and satisfied but you will also get an energy boost!

Serves: 1-2

Ingredients

- 1 big avocado, washed and pitted
- 1 cup of almond milk,
- 2 teaspoons of flaxseed meal
- A handful of fresh baby spinach, washed
- Optional: 1 teaspoon fresh moringa powder
- Optional: half cup filtered water or coconut water, if needed

Instructions
1. Place all ingredients in a blender.
2. Blend until combined and almonds are blitzed.
3. Serve into a chilled glass and enjoy!

Recipe#17 Spice Up Your Health Smoothie

This smoothie is perfect as a quick lunch or whenever you need an energy boost.

Oh, and it's spicy!

Serves:1-2

Ingredients

- 1 cup coconut milk
- chopped
- ½ cup of fresh green bell pepper, washed and chopped
- Half an avocado, peeled and pitted
- A pinch of chili powder
- 2 tablespoons of coconut oil
- A handful of fresh arugula leaves
- 1 tablespoon chia seeds
- Himalaya salt to taste

Instructions

1. Place all the ingredients in a blender.
2. Process until smooth.
3. Season with Himalayan salt to taste.
4. Serve and enjoy!

Recipe#18 The Anti-Age Smoothie

Dubbed "the beauty food", watercress is the secret weapon in this green machine, protein-packed smoothie. Watercress is the leader of anti-aging vegetables, with enormous amounts of vitamin K and other healthy nutrients that contribute to healthy skin, hair and nails.

Serves: 2-3

Ingredients

- ½ cup spinach
- 1 cucumber, chopped
- ½ cup of celery, chopped
- ½ cup of fresh watercress
- 2 cups of cashew or coconut milk
- 1 tablespoon coconut milk
- Pinch of Himalayan salt to taste, if needed

Instructions

1. Add all ingredients to a blender.
2. Processed well until smooth.
3. Enjoy!

Recipe#19 Refreshing Radish Green Smoothie

Radishes are very alkalizing and good for your liver and immune system. They are also very refreshing!

Servings: 1-2

Ingredients:

- Half cup radish, washed
- 1 small avocado, peeled and pitted
- A handful of fresh arugula leaves (or other greens of your choice)
- 1 cup full-fat coconut milk (no added sugar)
- Half cup of water, filtered, preferably alkaline
- Pinch of Himalaya salt to taste
- Pinch of black pepper to taste
- Optional: red chili pepper

Instructions:

1. Blend all the ingredients.
2. Serve in a smoothie glass or in a soup bowl- this smoothie can also be turned into a delicious soup.

Recipe#20 Cilantro Oriental Alkaline Keto Smoothie

Cilantro is a miraculous alkaline herb with potent antioxidant properties. It tastes great in smoothies, and so does curry powder!

Servings: 2-3

Ingredients:

- 2 cups coconut or almond milk
- 1 tablespoon coconut oil
- A handful of fresh cilantro leaves
- 1 small green bell pepper, sliced and seeded
- 1 teaspoon curry powder
- Pinch of Himalaya salt to taste
- Pinch of black pepper powder to taste
- Optional: a few drops of liquid chlorophyll

Instructions:

1. Combine all the ingredients in a blender.
2. Process until smooth.
3. Taste to check if you need to add more salt or spices.
4. Pour into a smoothie glass or a small soup bowl and enjoy!

Recipe#21 Vitamin C Alkaline Keto Green Power

This delicious smoothie is jam-packed with vitamin C coming from alkaline and keto friendly fruits like limes and lemons. Now, I understand that looking at the ingredients of this recipe, you may be feeling a bit "turned off." Yes, alkaline keto smoothies are very different to usual "sweet fruity smoothies."

But, give it a try. It tastes great! Very similar to natural, Greek yogurt. You can also use this smoothie recipe to season your salads. Most salad seasonings are full of crappy carbs, sugars and a ton of chemicals, while this smoothie is 100% natural! Another suggestion is - you could use this smoothie recipe to make a smoothie bowl by adding in some nuts and seeds. Once you have tried this smoothie, you will get my point for sure!

Servings: 2

Ingredients:

- 1 big avocado, peeled, pitted and sliced
- A small handful of spinach leaves
- Half lemon, peeled and sliced
- 1 cup of coconut milk
- 1 teaspoon coconut oil
- Pinch of Himalaya salt
- Pinch of black pepper
- A few slices of lime to garnish

Instructions:

1. Place all the ingredients in a blender.
2. Process until smooth.
3. Serve in a smoothie glass and garnish with a few lime slices.
4. Drink to your health and enjoy!

Recipe#22 Green Mineral Comfort Smoothie Soup

This recipe can be used both as a smoothie as well as a soup.

Whenever I am pressed for time, I make it for dinner, to enjoy something warm and keep the raw leftovers to have a healthy green smoothie in the morning.

Servings: 1-2

Ingredients:

- 1 big cucumber, peeled
- 1 small avocado, peeled and pitted
- A handful of parsley
- A handful of cilantro
- 1 cup of thick coconut milk
- A handful of raw cashews or pistachios (peel removed)
- 1 tablespoon of olive oil
- Himalaya salt to taste
- 1 chili flake (optional)

Instructions:

1. Blend all the ingredients in a blender.
2. Serve raw as a smoothie, or heat it up (using low heat) and serve as a gentle, detox, comforting soup.
3. Enjoy!

Recipe#23 Green Fat Burner Smoothie

This recipe combines the best fat-burning ingredients ever, helps you concentrate for long hours while feeling lighter.

It's also great if you suffer from water retention. Personally, I love drinking this smoothie in the summer.

Servings: 2

Ingredients:

- 1 green tea teabag (or 1 teaspoon green tea powder)
- 1 horsetail infusion tea bag (or 1 teaspoon horsetail infusion powder)
- 1 cup of water
- 1 big avocado
- 1 big grapefruit
- Half cup of coconut milk
- 1 teaspoon cinnamon powder
- Stevia to sweeten

Instructions:

1. Boil 1 cup of water.
2. Add in the green tea and horsetail infusion.
3. Cover.
4. In the meantime, process the remaining ingredients in a blender.
5. Add in the cooled herbal infusion and process again.
6. If needed sweeten with stevia.
7. Serve chilled and enjoy!

Recipe#24 Massive Green Power Plants Smoothie

If you don't like spinach or kale, I highly recommend you try arugula leaves. They taste delicious, both in salads and smoothies.

Servings: 3-4

Ingredients:

- 1 cup arugula leaves, washed
- 1 small avocado, peeled, pitted and sliced
- 2 cucumbers, peeled and sliced
- 4 tablespoons fresh lemon juice
- 2 tablespoons olive oil
- 2 cups hazelnut milk (unsweetened)
- Himalaya salt and black pepper to taste

Instructions:

1. Place all the ingredients in a blender.
2. Process well until smooth.
3. Serve and enjoy!

Recipe#25 Easy Guacamole Smoothie

This smoothie can also be used as a dip to be served with some veggies.

It also makes a great meal replacement if you are pressed for time and are looking for an easy and nutritious meal.

Servings: 1-2

Ingredients:

- 2 tomatoes, sliced
- Half avocado, peeled and sliced
- A handful of arugula leaves
- 1 small garlic clove, peeled and minced
- 4 tablespoons lime juice
- Half cup water, filtered
- 2 tablespoons olive oil
- Himalaya salt and black pepper to taste

Instructions:

1. Place all the ingredients in a blender.
2. Process well until smooth.
3. Serve and enjoy!

Recipe#26 Cucumber Kale Alkaline Keto Smoothies

Avocado oil offers good fat to help you absorb the minerals and vitamins from this smoothie. Celery stalks are full of vitamins and minerals, including vitamin K, vitamin A, potassium, and folate. Personally, I love using hot habanero sauce in my veggie smoothies. Who said that all smoothies must be sweet?

Servings: 3-4
Ingredients:
- 1 lemon, peeled
- 3 celery stalks, chopped
- A couple dashes of hot habanero sauce
- a handful of kale, chopped
- 2 big cucumbers, peeled and chopped
- 2 tablespoons of avocado oil
- Himalaya salt to taste
- 1 cup of water (filtered or alkaline)
- 1 cup of organic tomato juice

Instructions:
1. Place all the ingredients in a blender.
2. Process well until smooth.
3. Serve and enjoy!

Recipe#27 Sexy Flavored Spinach Smoothie

While pure spinach smoothie can be a bit boring, this recipe is a bit different.
Add in some fresh ginger and mix it with coconut milk and oil, and you will fall in love with spinach smoothie!

Serves: 2
Ingredients:
- Half cup of baby spinach
- 2-inch ginger, peeled
- 2 tablespoons coconut oil
- 1 cup of coconut milk

Instructions:
1. Place all the ingredients in a blender.
2. Process well until smooth.
3. Serve and enjoy!

Recipe#28 Spicy Broccoli Smoothie

I love this smoothie on my detox days. While, my regular diet is a balanced, clean food diet with a ton of keto and alkaline friendly foods (and some mini cheats occasionally), once or twice a year I like to go on a little detox- a food cleanse where I eat only alkaline foods. Actually, I love it so much that now I do it twice a year. It's an excellent self-development experience, you get to release the toxins and old patterns to embrace the new energies and opportunities. Not to mention the weight loss and healthy glow!

If you would like to learn more about the cleanse I like to do, I highly recommend Yuri Elkaim's program. You can learn more about it on my website:

www.YourWellnessBooks.com/resources

Perhaps you feel like the constant sugar cravings you are getting are sabotaging your health and weight loss goals. I have been there. Luckily, after going through the program, everything has changed for me (in a positive way).

Now...back to our detox smoothie. Like most vegetable smoothies, it can also be turned into a delicious soup.

Servings: 2

Ingredients:

- 1 cup broccoli florets, steamed or lightly cooked
- 1 garlic clove, peeled
- 1 chili flake or a pinch of chili powder
- A pinch of nutmeg powder
- A pinch of curry powder
- 1 cup full fat coconut milk

Alkaline Keto Green Smoothie Recipes

- 2 tablespoons coconut oil, or flax seed oil
- A handful of chive, minced

Instructions:

1. Place all the ingredients except chive in a blender.
2. Process well until smooth.
3. If needed, warm it up and serve as a soup, with some fresh chive in it.
4. Enjoy!

Recipe#29 Bullet Proof Chai Tea Anti-Inflammatory Green Smoothie

This smoothie will help you boost your energy almost instantly. Aside from chai tea, full of spices and antioxidant ingredients, it uses ginger and turmeric- one of the best anti-inflammatory superfoods there are! It tastes oriental, mysterious, and delicious!

Servings: 1-2
Ingredients
- 1 cup chai tea, cooled down (use 1 tea bag per cup)
- Half cup coconut or almond milk (unsweetened)
- 1 tablespoon coconut oil
- A few drops of liquid chlorophyll
- Half avocado, peeled
- A handful of blueberries
- 1-inch ginger, peeled
- 1 teaspoon spirulina powder
- Half teaspoon turmeric powder
- Half teaspoon cinnamon powder to add on top

Instructions:
1. Blend all the ingredients (except cinnamon) using a blender.
2. Pour your smoothie into a smoothie glass and serve with ice cubes if needed.
3. Sprinkle some cinnamon powder on top. Enjoy!

Recipe#30 Easy and Tasty Green Smoothie Maravilla

Most people don't like green smoothies, because they haven't tried enough of them. And let's face it- a dull, annoying, spinach, or kale smoothie is not very appealing.

Luckily this one, doesn't taste gross!

Servings: 2
Ingredients
- 1 cup coconut, cashew or almond milk (unsweetened)
- Half cup water, filtered, preferably alkaline
- 1 tablespoon avocado oil or olive oil
- half cup fresh parsley leaves, washed
- half cup fresh cilantro leaves, washed
- pinch of Himalayan salt
- pinch of black pepper
- 1 teaspoon chia seeds
- A handful of cashews

Instructions:
1. Place all the ingredients in a blender.
2. Process until smooth.
3. Serve and enjoy!
4. If needed, add more salt and black pepper.

Suggestion- you can serve this smoothie as a quick, raw, nourishing soup. You can also add some fresh veggies or meal leftovers.

Recipe#31 Green Vegan Keto Smoothie for Weight Loss

This smoothie is rich in good fats, good protein, and healthy greens to help you lose weight and feel amazing. It's one of those smoothies that will help you reduce sugar cravings and stay full for hours!

Servings: 2
Ingredients
- 2 cup thick coconut milk (full fat)
- 2 tablespoons coconut oil
- Half avocado, peeled and sliced
- Half lemon, peeled and sliced
- 2 tablespoons fresh cilantro leaves
- Black pepper (optional)
- Himalayan salt

Instructions:
1. Place all the ingredients in a blender.
2. Process until smooth.
3. Serve and enjoy!
4. If needed, season with more black pepper and Himalayan salt.

Recipe#32 Quick Unwind Smoothie

This smoothie uses healing herbal infusions-rooibos. Rooibos is full of minerals such as Iron and Magnesium. Gluten-free oat milk is very healthy, and it has sleep-inducing properties. Avocado and coconut oil will help you prevent sugar cravings and sleep like a baby.

Servings: 2
Ingredients
- 1 cup rooibos tea (cooled down, use 1 teabag per cup)
- 1 cup gluten-free oat milk
- 1 teaspoon coconut oil
- 1 small avocado, peeled and pitted
- A small handful of baby spinach leaves
- 1 little lime, peeled and sliced
- A handful of cashews
- 1 teaspoon cinnamon powder
- Stevia to sweeten if needed

Instructions:
1. Place all the ingredients in a blender.
2. Process until smooth.
3. Enjoy now or place in a fridge for later.

Recipe#33 Spicy Mediterranean Protein Smoothie

This delicious veggie smoothie can also be served as a quick, raw soup. Perfect as a quick meal replacement or a quick, nourishing meal.

Servings: 2
Ingredients
- 1 cup almond milk, unsweetened
- 1 tablespoon extra-virgin olive oil
- 1 cup organic tomato juice
- 1 green bell pepper, chopped
- Half avocado, peeled
- Half cucumber, peeled
- A handful of cashews
- Himalayan salt to taste
- A pinch of black pepper
- A pinch of chili powder
- A few drops of liquid chlorophyll

Instructions:
1. Place all the ingredients in a blender.
2. Process until smooth, serve, and enjoy!

Recipe#34 Vitamin C Energy and Mood Boosting Smoothie

Having a bad day? Do you need to boost your mood? Try this smoothie. It offers a healthy mix of vitamin C, energy stimulating greens, and mood-boosting cocoa.

Servings: 1-2
Ingredients
- 1 cup coconut milk or gluten-free rice milk (unsweetened)
- Half cup water, filtered, preferably alkaline water
- 1 teaspoon coconut oil
- 1-inch ginger, peeled
- 1-inch turmeric, peeled
- Half cup arugula leaves
- 1 grapefruit, peeled
- Stevia to sweeten (optional)
- Half teaspoon cinnamon
- 1 tablespoon cocoa powder
- 1 tablespoon chia seeds
- A few drops of liquid chlorophyll

Instructions:
1. Blend and enjoy.
2. Add some stevia to sweeten if needed.
3. This drink is great first thing in the morning. But you can also sip on it during the day to enjoy more energy or whenever you are having a bad day!

Recipe#35 Green Almond Protein Hormone Balancer

This delicious smoothie uses maca powder, which is a hormone re-balancer for women.

Servings: 1-2
Ingredients
- 1 cup coconut or almond milk (unsweetened)
- 1 tablespoon coconut oil
- Half cup coconut water
- Half cup kale leaves
- 1 avocado, peeled and pitted
- Half green apple
- A bit of stevia to sweeten
- Half teaspoon fresh maca powder
- 1 tablespoon hemp seed protein powder (personally, I like chocolate-flavored protein powder)

+ a few lime slices and ice cubes to serve if needed

Instructions:
1. Place all the ingredients in a blender.
2. Process until smooth.
3. Serve and enjoy!
4. This smoothie also tastes delicious when chilled or half-frozen.

Recipe #36 Creamy Alkaline Smoothie Refresher

The smoothie is naturally creamy and very tasty. The cinnamon powder makes this smoothie nice and sweet. Coconut oil will help you reduce sugar cravings.

Serves: 1-2
Ingredients
- 2 cups cold coconut milk, unsweetened
- 1 tablespoon coconut oil
- 2 tablespoons fresh lime juice
- 1 small avocado, peeled and pitted
- A handful of cashews, raw, soaked in filtered water for at least a few hours
- A few basil leaves
- A few mint leaves
- 1 tablespoon chia seeds
- 1 teaspoon cinnamon powder
- Half teaspoon ginger powder
- Optional- stevia to sweeten

Instructions
1. Blend all the ingredients using a blender.
2. Process until smooth.
3. Serve and enjoy! This nutritious smoothie makes a great breakfast.

Recipe#37 Alkaline Keto Fill Me Up Smoothie

This alkaline-vegan smoothie tastes a bit like Greek yogurt but is entirely plant-based and dairy-free.

Serves: 1-2
Ingredients
Liquid:
- 2 cups cold unsweetened almond milk
- 1 tablespoon avocado oil
- 2 tablespoons chia seeds (or chia seed powder)
- 1 small lemon, peeled and sliced
- 1 small avocado, peeled and pitted
- A few drops of liquid chlorophyll
- a few lime slices to garnish
- a pinch of Himalayan salt
- a pinch of black pepper to taste

Instructions
1. Place all the ingredients in a blender.
2. Blend until smooth. Serve and enjoy!

Recipe#38 Holistic Beauty Smoothie

This alkaline vegan smoothie is designed to help you have a super healthy-looking, glowing skin while increasing your energy levels at the same time!

Serves: 1-2
Ingredients
- 1 cup cashew milk
- Half cup of coconut water
- 2 small carrots, peeled
- 1 big green bell pepper, cut into smaller pieces
- 2 tablespoons chia seeds
- 1 teaspoon cinnamon powder
- A few drops of liquid cinnamon
- stevia to sweeten if needed
- fresh mint leaves and lime slices to serve

Instructions
1. Place all the ingredients in a blender.
2. Blend until smooth.
3. Pour into a glass and enjoy!

Recipe#39 Heal Up Smoothie

If you want to transition to making super healthy alkaline vegan smoothies, you gotta explore moringa, mint, and cilantro! Moringa is a natural protein alkaline superfood. It contains all the essential amino acids – the building blocks of protein- that are needed to grow, repair, and maintain cells. At the same time, it's rich in alkaline-forming minerals such as magnesium, iron, and potassium.

Serves: 1-2
Ingredients
- 1 cup of coconut milk
- Half cup fresh grapefruit juice
- Handful almonds, soaked in filtered water for at least a few hours
- 1-inch fresh ginger, peeled
- A few avocado slices
- 1 teaspoon moringa powder
- A handful of fresh mint washed
- A handful of fresh cilantro leaves washed

Instructions
1. Place all the ingredients into a blender
2. Process well until smooth. Enjoy!

Recipe#40 Create Massive Balance Alkaline Smoothie

This smoothie is perfect as a quick detox smoothie to help you enjoy more energy!

Servings: 2-3
Ingredients
- 1 cup almond milk
- Half cup water, filtered, preferably alkaline
- 1 tablespoon coconut oil
- 2 big cucumbers, peeled and roughly sliced
- 1 big avocado
- Half lemon, peeled and sliced
- 4 tablespoons almonds, chopped or powdered
- A handful of cilantro
- 1 tablespoon almond or hemp seed protein powder
- Pinch of Himalaya salt to taste
- Pinch of black pepper to taste
- 2 tablespoons chive, chopped
- 1 teaspoon spirulina powder

Instructions:
1. Place all the ingredients in a blender.
2. Blend well and pour into a smoothie glass or a small soup bowl.
3. Serve and enjoy!

Recipe#41 Simple Detox Spicy Smoothie

If you are looking for a quick detox recipe-this smoothie recipe will help you sweat out all the toxins and supercharge your nutrition!

Servings: 2-3
Ingredients
- 1 cup organic tomato juice
- Half cup unsweetened almond milk
- 2 big cucumbers, peeled and roughly sliced
- 6 radishes, sliced
- 2 tablespoons chive, chopped
- 1 garlic clove, peeled
- Half cup arugula leaves, washed
- 1 teaspoon hemp protein powder
- Pinch of Himalayan salt
- Pinch of black pepper
- Pinch of chili powder

Instructions:
1. Place all the ingredients through a blender.
2. Blend, serve, and enjoy!
3. You can also serve this smoothie as a quick, raw detox soup.

Recipe#42 Ultimate Wellness Alkaline Green Smoothie

This smoothie tastes delicious, and I highly recommend it for days where your goal is detoxification to have more energy.

Servings: 2-3
Ingredients
- 1 cup coconut or almond milk
- Half cup water, filtered, preferably alkaline
- 1 tablespoon coconut oil
- 2 big cucumbers, peeled and roughly sliced
- 1 big avocado
- Half lemon, peeled and sliced
- 4 tablespoons almonds, chopped or powdered
- A handful of cilantro
- 1 tablespoon chia seeds
- Pinch of Himalaya salt to taste
- Pinch of black pepper to taste
- 2 tablespoons chive, chopped
- 1 teaspoon spirulina powder

Instructions:
1. Place all the ingredients in a blender.
2. Blend well and pour into a smoothie glass or a small soup bowl.
3. Serve and enjoy!

Recipe#43 Liver Cleanse Green Smoothie

If you want to improve your energy levels, consider doing a mini liver cleanse. One of the ways I like to go about it is to start my day with 2 glasses of warm water (preferably alkaline) with 2 tablespoons of lemon juice.

Then, I have this smoothie for breakfast. The rest of my diet remains very clean (lots of veggies, organic foods, no gluten, no dairy, no alcohol), and I stick with it for 2 weeks (usually during springtime).

Servings: 1-2
Ingredients
- 1 cup full-fat coconut milk (no added sugar)
- Half cup of water, filtered, preferably alkaline
- Half cup radish washed
- 1 small avocado, peeled and pitted
- A handful of fresh arugula leaves
- Pinch of Himalaya salt to taste
- 1 teaspoon chlorella
- 1 teaspoon spirulina
- 1 teaspoon chia seeds

Instructions:
1. Blend all the ingredients.
2. Serve in a smoothie glass or in a soup bowl- this smoothie can also be turned into a delicious soup.

Recipe#44 Super Antioxidant Green Smoothie

Cilantro is a miraculous alkaline herb with potent antioxidant properties. It tastes great in smoothies!

Especially when backed up with creamy nut milk and some spices and superfoods to help you thrive!

Sometimes, I like to have this smoothie for breakfast, especially when I am tired and need to restore my energy quickly.

My ritual is- have this smoothie as a quick, early dinner, relax, meditate, and have an early night.

The next day, I feel like a new person, all because of the balancing and antioxidant properties of this smoothie.

I also highly recommend you look into Ashwagandha, it truly is a miraculous herb.

I have written an entire book on Ashwagandha if you are interested in diving deeper (www.amazon.com/author/elenagarcia)

Servings: 2-3
Ingredients
Liquid:
- 2 cups gluten-free oat milk (or any other plant-based milk)
- 1 tablespoon coconut oil
- A handful of fresh cilantro leaves
- 2 small carrots, peeled
- 1 teaspoon chlorella
- Half teaspoon Ashwagandha

- 1 teaspoon moringa
- Half teaspoon cinnamon powder
- Pinch of Himalaya salt to taste

Instructions:
1. Combine all the ingredients in a blender.
2. Process until smooth.
3. Taste to check if you need to add some Himalayan salt or spices.
4. Pour into a smoothie glass or a small soup bowl and enjoy it!

Alkaline Keto Green Smoothie Recipes

Recipe#45 Keto Fill Me Up Smoothie

This smoothie is rich in good fats and very low in carbs. At the same time, it incorporates a myriad of different nutrient-packed superfoods. The perfect recipe to fill you up and help you stay energized for hours.

Servings: 2
Ingredients
- 1 cup of coconut milk
- Half cup cashew milk
- 2 teaspoons olive oil
- 1 big avocado, peeled, pitted and sliced
- Half lemon, peeled and sliced
- A handful of cashews
- A handful of almonds
- 1 teaspoon spirulina
- 1 teaspoon chlorella
- Himalayan salt to taste

Instructions:
1. Place all the ingredients in a blender.
2. Process until smooth.
3. Serve in a smoothie glass and garnish with a few lime slices.
4. Drink to your health, and enjoy it!

Recipe#46 Hormone Rebalancer Sweet Veggie Smoothie

This smoothie is naturally sweet even though it doesn't use any fruit. It's because red bell peppers are naturally delicious veggies. Then, coconut water adds in a more natural sweet taste, while stevia and cinnamon take it to the next level.

Moringa and spirulina not only add some natural protein but also turn this smoothie into a green, chlorophyll-rich, nourishing smoothie.

Servings: 1-2
Ingredients
Liquid:

- 2 cups of coconut water
- 1 tablespoon coconut oil
- 1 big red bell pepper
- 2 medium-size carrots, peeled
- Half avocado, peeled and sliced
- Half teaspoon moringa powder
- Half teaspoon spirulina powder
- Half teaspoon cinnamon powder
- Stevia to sweeten, if needed

Instructions:
1. Blend all the ingredients in a blender.
2. Serve and enjoy!

Questions?

You can email me at:

info@yourwellnessbooks.com

Alkaline Ketogenic Smoothies is the second book in the Alkaline Keto Diet Book series.

The first book in the series is called: *Alkaline Ketogenic Mix*: *Quick, Easy, and Delicious Recipes & Tips for Natural Weight Loss and a Healthy Lifestyle.*
It's a step-by-step beginner guide to help you transition to a healthy alkaline-keto way of eating without feeling deprived.

You will find all the Alkaline Keto Diet books on Amazon & listed on our website:

www.amazon.com/author/elenagarcia

www.yourwellnessbooks.com/books

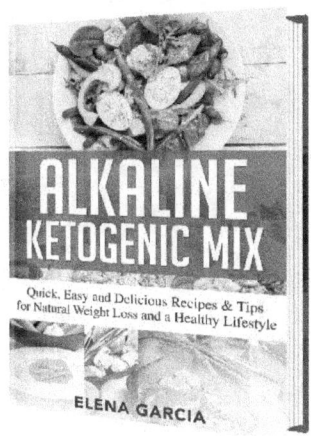

Extra Resources to Help You on Your Journey

I am regularly updating my website with new health and wellness recommendations (books, resources, natural supplements, and products).

My purpose and mission is to help you with easy-to-follow guides while sharing what has worked for me on my journey.

The goal is to keep it very simple, doable, and fun to help you enjoy vibrant health and, if desired, start losing weight (naturally).

Wellness doesn't have to be complicated or expensive. Quite on the contrary.

What matters is the actions you decide to take right here, right now. Little, imperfect but meaningful actions will lead you to beautiful results as the compound effect will start taking place.

Thank you again for reading.

I am really grateful for you,

Until next time,

Wishing you all the best on your journey,

Elena

We Need Your Help

One more thing, before you go, could you please do us a quick favor?

It would be great if you could leave us a short review online.

Don't worry, it doesn't have to be long. One sentence is enough.

Let others know your favorite recipes and who you think this book can help.

Many people drink "normal" smoothies and don't even realize they are overdoing sugar and carbs. No wonder they give up...

Your review can inspire more and more people to turn to low-carb, low-sugar nutrient-packed smoothies so that they can finally achieve their wellness and weight loss goals the way they deserve.

Your honest review is critical.

Thank You for your support!

Join Our VIP Readers' Newsletter to Boost Your Wellbeing

Would you like to be notified about our new health and wellness books?

How about receiving them at deeply discounted prices? And before anyone else?

What about awesome giveaways, latest health tips, and motivation?

If that is something you are interested in, please visit the link below to join our newsletter:

www.yourwellnessbooks.com/email-newsletter

It's 100% free + spam free (we hate spam as much as you do)

We promise we will only email you with valuable and relevant information, delicious recipes, and tips to help you on your journey.

Sign up link:

www.yourwellnessbooks.com/email-newsletter

More Books & Resources in the Healthy Lifestyle Series

Available at:

www.yourwellnessbooks.com

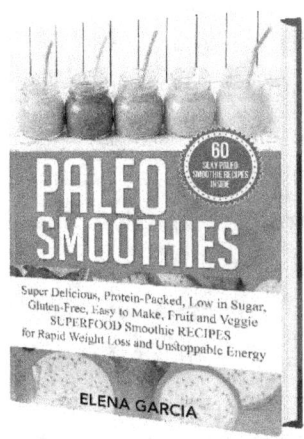
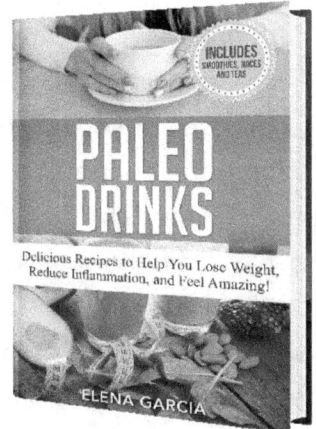
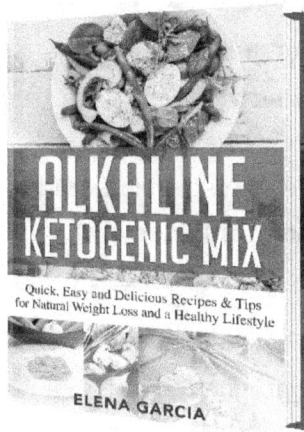
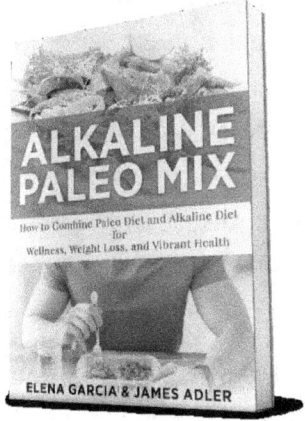

A physician has not written the information in this book. It is advisable that you visit a qualified dietician so that you can obtain a highly personalized treatment for your case, especially if you want to lose weight effectively. This book is for informational and educational purposes only and is not intended for medical purposes. Please consult your physician before making any drastic changes to your diet.

All information in this book has been carefully researched and checked for factual accuracy. However, the author and publishers make no warranty, expressed or implied, that the information contained herein is appropriate for every individual, situation or purpose, and assume no responsibility for errors or omission. The reader assumes the risk, and full responsibility for all actions and the author will not be held liable for any loss or damage, whether consequential, incidental, and special or otherwise, that may result from the information presented in this publication.

The book is not intended to provide medical advice or to take the place of medical advice and treatment from your personal physician. Readers are advised to consult their own doctors or other qualified health professionals regarding the treatment of medical conditions. The author shall not be held liable or responsible for any misunderstanding or misuse of the information contained in this book. The information is not intended to diagnose, treat, or cure any disease.

If you suffer from any medical condition, are pregnant, lactating, or on medication, be sure to talk to your doctor before making any drastic changes in your diet and lifestyle.

www.ingramcontent.com/pod-product-compliance
Lightning Source LLC
Chambersburg PA
CBHW071750080526
44588CB00013B/2202